GRATEFUL *for an* UNLIKELY GIFT

A Message of Divine Hope
on
My Personal Journey with Cancer

by

Japonica Walker

PLEASE NOTE THAT *GRATEFUL FOR AN UNLIKELY GIFT* IS A MEMOIR AND REFLECTS ONLY THE PERSONAL EXPERIENCE AND VIEWS OF THE AUTHOR. The ideas and suggestions herein are my own experiences. There may be some ideas in the book that may not agree with orthodox, allopathic medicine.

NOTE: The information contained in this book is for educational purposes only. The medical conditions discussed in this book should only be under the direction of a physician. Proper care from a physician should not be avoided, delayed, or discarded when there's a reason to consult a physician. This book isn't designed to diagnose, treat, or recommend a particular therapy. The author accepts no responsibility for such use. Conditions requiring proper medical attention should be referred to a physician. JAPONICA WALKER

Published in the United States by TDR Brands Publishing

Dedication

This book is dedicated to My Jesus, who taught me how to truly live when threatened with a diagnosis of breast cancer.

A thief comes only to steal and kill and destroy. I have come so they may have life. I want them to have it in the fullest possible way.
(John 10:10 NIRV)

Acknowledgments

To my body, which has been fearfully and wonderfully made by My Jesus. It has been the greatest teacher in knowing my Savior. It has taught me that God has paid a great price for me to live a whole and prosperous life by honoring Him. I am a priority to Him and have great value.

To my dear friend Nola, who was a true friend and sister in every sense of the word, every step of the way. She was the very embodiment of Our Lord. No matter how dark the times got or how ugly I acted, she loved me through it. My angel!

To my awesome husband, who rallied the family together as a unit to financially support my decision to go to Optimum Health Institute. He was my rock, even though he was afraid too. We came together and worked as one. This God opportunity caused him to press into our Lord as well. Anything that causes us to get in God's face is a good thing.

To my beautiful children, who financially backed me to go down to the Optimum Health Institute for a natural and holistic approach to health. They made it happen!

To Mrs. Warfield, who was one of the best cheerleaders and promoters in the world, for her patience and unending effort in helping conceptualize this book. She believed in me, every step of the way. She dedicated her time, talents, and skills to help carry out God's purpose in writing this book.

To my loving mom, who loved me, supported me, praised me, told me continually how proud of me she was and how glad she was that I chose to follow God's instructions concerning the natural way of healing.

To Mrs. Gaines, who pointed me to Dr. Waggoner, a medical doctor, who believe there was another way to approach cancer.

To Dr. Jill Waggoner, who was a vital team member, from the medical perspective, who supported and honored my decision to go the holistic route.

To Mrs. McCray, who prayed for me continuously and made me feel valuable.

Words From an Angel!

I've known Japonica (Rena) since the beginning of time! Well, actually, we've known each other for 20+ years. She is the sister of my heart.

We met at Langley Air Force Base Fitness Center where we were fitness instructors. Our husbands were career military. I knew right away that she was a person I'd love to call friend. We've gone through good and bad times to together.

When she asked me to write this foreword, I felt honored. Journeying with her as she battled cancer was frightening! I was afraid of losing her, of not having her to laugh with, to be real with, or to rein me in when I believed God had spoken a word to me and I'd take off running. Whenever I would start to run, Japonica would ask: "Did you get the details? "Did you ask questions?" Then she'd say, "Wait for God to put skin on it!"

My relationship with God has gone to a deeper level through sharing this journey with her. All my life, I've heard "God will never give you more than you can handle," and never doubted it. But, during that time, I began to question its veracity! I vowed to myself to be to her what Aaron was to Moses in Exodus 17:10–12. I would walk beside her and hold up her arms when she got tired and to pray for her without ceasing. Having gone through this experience with Japonica, I've come to believe the statement about God never giving us more than we can handle to be true.

Japonica is one AWESOME woman. I thank God for bringing her into my life and allowing me to walk beside her!

Inola Garrett

Table of Contents

A Special Note

A Husband's Perspective

It's important to me to first share how we met and why I believe this marriage has lasted over 35 years. I met Japonica while we were both stationed at Osan Air Base, Korea in January of 1983. We were married in July of the same year. How did this happen? I was young, single, handsome, and full of myself. I certainly wasn't looking for a wife. We attended the base Chapel and were part of the base Choir where she sung. I just thought I could. At the time, I had a pre-Christian belief that no man could stay married to one women for the rest of his life and remain faithful. Even then, divorce was just as prevalent in the church as it was in the world.

One night, in ignorance, I prayed this prayer, "Lord Jesus if I get married I want my wife to be a seven-day-a-week Christian, someone after your Heart, not a Sunday Christian." I had dated many Sunday Christian women in my life. I had no idea if God had heard me, and went about my day-to-day activities as a good churchgoer. We weren't dating at the time. Then, some weeks later, God answered me through a very real dream and vision that Japonica was to be my wife.

Of all the doubts and concerns I've had about God speaking to me, one thing I've never doubted is that Japonica is exactly the woman I prayed for; though, at the time of the prayer, I didn't know what that would look like. Never have I wanted to leave the marriage, even though I used to tell some of my work associates that if I were her, I would have left me a long time ago. This was mostly because of my extensive travels and time away while she was carrying all the responsibilities. I no longer use those words. And now I really understand why she may have felt like leaving.

When I found out about my wife's diagnosis it was like being hit with a ton of bricks full of fear, anger, confusion, and tears. This is the woman I knew God had brought into my life. I was angry, very angry, confused and wanted to know why this happened to her. Also, at times, I would be the tempter to test what she shared about what God had asked her to do. Admittedly, I even had the nerve to get jealous because he didn't tell me first. Now, I realize that maybe I wasn't listening.

One of the hardest things for her to do was to surrender her womb. She gave up a promising military career to raise our family. She also homeschooled our eight kids.

I was and, still to this day, am angry at God for allowing this. It certainly doesn't seem fair, good, or just. Her labor in the Lord, at times, seems to have been in vain and unrewarded. Somewhere deep inside of me, I don't believe her labor was in vain.

Even though we were both Christians, our different perspectives was one reason we had so many areas of disagreement. My own stubbornness was another reason. I have fought against, and not fully supported, her in all the hard paths she has been placed on. Each hard path where she sacrificed her way for His way only confirmed that I got what I asked the Lord for when I prayed for a wife who was not just a Sunday Christian, but a seven-day-a week Christian. But, I've never doubted that God provided exactly the woman I prayed for, and needed.

I really don't believe I would be here today without her. I don't understand God's reward system, but it didn't seem to apply to my wife. I know that there's always some light in darkness and am still awaiting to see the light in her case.

I know that real Love is not "pie in the sky." It's real when you can feel it, when you walk together, cry together, mourn together, sacrifice together, play together, laugh together, rejoice together, and pray together. I've struggled in the way I have loved my wife. One night while praying about our relationship, healing, and how to love her in this hard place, God impressed on my spirit to Love her with the love she can feel.

Her sharing her heart about the greatness she feels inside and her fear that she will die with her greatness inside confirms even more this is the women God put in my life. I now realize the risk of marriage. It's worth whatever it cost and more, if it's from God's perspective.

My heart's desire and prayer is for my wife's season of greatness to be realized to all and manifested in whatever medium God chooses.

Introduction

Wow! It has been a journey! I remember when I first got the cancer diagnosis. I was filled with fear, anxiety, crying, and the last emotions were ones of anger and fury! Was it possible that after 30 years of serving the Lord that my life was going to end up being ravaged by cancer? It was extremely hard to wrap my mind around that idea. "Where is God in all this?" I repeatedly asked!

The purpose of this book is to instill hope into the reader. Regardless of the path chosen to confront life's sometimes overwhelming challenges and problems, God can give His hope. He is our Divine Hope. This Divine Hope does not assure us of the outcomes we desire. However, it assures us that, regardless of the outcome, Jesus Christ is with us every step of the way. This hope is the "LIGHT" for our paths when it feels like our lives are in complete and utter darkness (Ps. 119:105).

This story is about how the diagnosis of breast cancer became an opportunity to trust in the Lord Jesus Christ. Was it scary? Yes, but it was certainly worth it! It was one of few times for me that it was easier to trust God than my own human reasoning. I felt like I didn't have very many options. The thought of the conventional way of treating cancer and all the horrific stories I was told by others caused me to run to my Lord for answers on what I needed to do with this new "challenge."

As a big proponent of practicality in my life, I was willing to do what was needed physically, spiritually, and nutritionally for complete healing. However, I needed some Supernatural directions! After unsuccessfully consulting numerous medical professionals, I decided, on my own, to gather the information needed to make a sound and wise decision that would work best for me and my family. As I walked out of the office of the second oncologist, feeling enraged at the thought that no one could offer me a guarantee, I received a "Divine Download" on my next steps. I began to feel hopeful that God had heard my grumblings.

After many prayers and gathering information on the best possible solutions that would guarantee I would not die, and weighing the pros and cons of conventional therapies versus natural therapies, I concluded that His Will for my life was to seek natural therapies and trust Him for the answers. With my family, I made the decision to take the first steps toward trusting God in the process. I was terrified; however, God proved to be faithful! We decided that Optimum Health Institute (OHI) was the place where we would learn to trust God with this health crisis. At this holistic center, God began to unveil the root causes of the breast cancer. Now tell me! How many people realize that most diseases have some kind of emotional root? We hear the word *cancer,* and we immediately run to the doctors for a solution, and not to our God.

I so desperately needed God's perspective on this situation; but, I have since discovered that Heaven's perspective is needed in my life every single day. It was and is His perspective that brings me life, hope, and dispels fear and anxiety. This began a time of consecration to the Lord during which the Lord's Prayer became meaningful and practical. Consider this idea! Our problems are a platform to praise our God. The act of praise creates the environment to hear God's perspective on the problem. So why do we resist the problems that come into our lives? His heavenly perspective brought me the wonderful gift of peace. I have grown addicted to this kind of peace. This is the peace of God that surpasses all human understanding (Phil. 4:7). When we have peace, we seem to make better decisions that will impact our future and our families. Once the peace was there, I was in a position to obtain enough of God's Plan to move in His purpose through the problem.

That was a tongue twister! Did you catch it? His plan, oh my God, caused me to approach problems not as obstacles, but as opportunities.

Don't be mistaken! This was a very tough journey of trusting in the God who I proclaimed was my Lord, my All in All, My Rock, and the list can go on and on. It's easier to say than to actually live out! Here was a perfect opportunity to get to know Him as all those things that I had so ignorantly and so arrogantly proclaimed. It was time to replace my fear with faith. There's no way I could have done this without having a personal relationship with God in which He was and is truly involved in speaking into my life. In walking this journey, His words out of His mouth to my ears gave me the courage to travel this <u>hellacious</u> path. Understand, this was a very intimate word from God to me. This kind of journey, in my opinion, requires your faith to speak to you personally!

After 18 months of working with Dr. Waggoner and working with a variety of natural therapies, we were able to bring the cancer markers back to normal range. Dr. Waggoner, my family, friends and I were elated at the results! We celebrated my healing!

Following His Plan exposed His provisions. His plan revealed many areas in which I had offended and disrespected my God, myself, and others. His pardon for my ignorance was magnificent! I had a lot of repenting to do. To behold how God had protected me was unbelievable! He protected me from sin, self, and Satan. That's the unholy trinity! Therefore, I've been commissioned to proclaim His mighty acts of power! To Him be the glory, the honor, and the power, forever. Amen.

CHAPTER I

God, I Wrecked My Mercedes Benz!

I t's so easy for Christians to ignorantly pray to the God of the universe and ask for things without knowing the cost. What makes us think that the Omnipotent God thinks like mere humans when it comes to matters of the heart, life, or death?

Years ago, I remember praying to know the Lord Jesus in the power of His Resurrection, the fellowship of his sufferings, being made conformable to His death (Phil. 3:10). Doesn't it sound really pious and spiritual? Little did I know that God not only heard me, but also had a plan to answer that prayer for His glory—not for my own glory! He certainly didn't answer in a way that I would have chosen.

God loves people and He cares about how they suffer. Christ suffered so that He would be able to identify with us as humans, and provide a solution to our problems. A solution that would be beneficial not only to us personally, but also to others. God bears witness to this in 2 Corinthians 1:3–7:

> *Blessed be God, even the Father of our Lord Jesus Christ, the Father of mercies, and the God of all comfort; Who comforted us in all our tribulation, that we may be able to comfort them which are in any trouble, by the comfort wherewith we ourselves are comforted of God. For as the sufferings of Christ abound in us, so our consolation also abounded by Christ. And whether we be afflicted, It's for your consolation and salvation, which is effectual in the enduring of the same sufferings which we also suffer: or whether we be comforted, It's for your consolation and salvation. And our hope of you is steadfast, knowing, that as ye are partakers of the sufferings, so shall ye be also of the consolation.*

He left us His Holy Spirit so that we would follow His example. Nobody wants to hear about how to suffer as Christ did. Why don't we want to look at righteous suffering as an opportunity to emulate Christ? I sure didn't! Do you?

You've heard of the saying, "Be careful what you ask for; you just might get it." What seemed like the end of an intense spiritual obedience training session was only the beginning of what was to come.

For years, I'd had problems with my digestive system. I would soon learn that my bad nutritional choices; a disrespect for my body, emotions, and spirit; and my unrealistic expectations would only make matters worse. I found out from my mother that a weakened digestive system ran in our family. No one in my family had prepared me for the gut and health issues that I would experience

Up until the age of 30, I had pretty much lived my life on my own terms, even though I was a Christian. At the time, I really didn't have a good reason to change the way I was living. I wasn't happy in my marriage, but I was okay. I lived this way not out of arrogance, but out of ignorance. God certainly didn't call the shots when it came to what I put in my mouth, or how I handled myself in relationships. I didn't know that He cared, nor did I know that the way that I was living was destructive. I was an avid churchgoer. I went to church every Sunday and sang in the choir. I gave tithes and offerings. I participated in Bible study on Wednesday nights. I read my Bible. I prayed daily. However, I felt that something was still missing. I couldn't quite put my finger on it.

I began to ask God to draw my husband and me closer. I began to seek God for answers. I had a new baby, but my husband and I were constantly arguing. Finances were low. I felt like a single military parent who was home-schooling while my husband was away. I was begging God to DO SOME-THING! You know that kind of prayer when you say, "Lord, whatever you say I'll do it!" I didn't have a clue!

Boy, was I clueless about what I was asking God for. Well, let me go a little deeper for you. In January of 1990, I had my fifth child after a devastating miscarriage. I was excited about having a new baby. I got sheer joy in naming him Emanuel, God with us! I was 29 years old when Emanuel was born, and I was excited about my upcoming 30th birthday in June. I had no idea that my life was about to change in a way that I would not have imagined.

It was June 7th. My birthday comes and goes, and life is good. Or is it? Stress is at an all-time high. One day, my family and I were having lunch at the military base club house in Germany. I began to eat a steamed carrot, and it got lodged in my throat. A panic came over me like no other. I thought I was going to die! I couldn't breathe; I couldn't talk. I panicked and quickly ran to the restroom. Sweat was pouring off of me like I had been running a marathon. I didn't know what was happening. My husband was standing outside of the bathroom door begging me to let him help me. He was shouting, "Honey, are you alright?" All I could do, in my mind, was cry out to the Lord. "Lord Jesus, please help me!" After a few minutes of shear dread, the carrot finally passed through the esophagus. This was my first encounter with what seemed to be death. Little did I know that my body and my health were demanding a change. It helped me to realize how valuable it was to be able to swallow. I had taken the power to swallow for granted. This was one of my many repentances; I begged God to forgive me! I later found out that I had a problem with listening to what God had to say about my life.

That episode with the carrot made me cautious about what I put in mouth. Unfortunately for me, the change only lasted for a short time. The next encounter with "the agent of change" was when I was drinking a glass of water and it had the same effect on my body as the carrot did. I couldn't swallow the water! It was as if my throat had closed shut. Panic quickly set in again! Of course, as a spirit-filled, evangelical, go-to-church-every-time-the-doors-open Christian, I had to pull out my Rebuker! The encounter with water took a little bit longer to swallow than the carrot. Can you believe that? After this episode ended, I began to ask God what was going on. It was simply water! How hard could it be to swallow water? Jesus, help me!

After several incidences of food and liquids getting lodged, I became fearful at meal times. I was desperate for an answer. I had babies to raise. Surely, God didn't intend for me to die right now! Did He? What was going to happen to my babies if I passed away? I sought out medical attention on several occasions. Eventually, I was diagnosed with a debilitating hiatal hernia. This was a condition in which the colon was severely inflamed, and the inflammation caused the whole digestive tract to push upwards. It was my body's way of talking to me and attempting to get me to change my lifestyle habits (I know that now, but not then). The military doctors (we were in Germany at the time of the diagnosis) told me that there was nothing that they could do about the hiatal hernia. I felt hopeless. My children were babies! I begged

God for mercy to allow me to see my babies grow up. He was merciful, but instructed me that I would have to change how I was living and how I was taking care of myself. So began the journey to holistic nutrition and balanced living. This would be one of many severe health "opportunities" that I would encounter on this journey toward the purposes of God.

Over the next 20 years, my digestive system served as a constant reminder that I had to treat it with a great deal of respect; otherwise, things would not go well with me. If the gut isn't right, you can't take a bite! If you can't nourish your body properly, life becomes limited, scary, and very uncomfortable. If you can't move your bowels (taking the trash out), the body (the house) becomes filled with toxic waste. Picture this: you have 10 one-gallon bags of trash in your house and you can't take it out. Each week the trash just continues to pile up in the house! Can you imagine the smell?

One day, about seven years ago, I noticed a black lump on my lower back. It looked like I had been hit in the back with a hard object. It was tender, but I wasn't in pain. It looked quite unusual. I had been working so hard (or so I thought) to show my digestive system respect. I didn't realize at that time that my emotions were completely unhealthy and contributed to my digestive malfunctions. I used all kinds of conventional, as well as natural, ways to keep my bowels moving.

Many people don't realize how important gut health is to their overall well-being. The digestive system is considered in traditional naturopathy and in certain medical communities to be the "second brain" of the human system.

The gut is constantly communicating with the brain about what nutrients from foods and drinks are acceptable and which ones are not. The digestive system is considered to be important in breaking down whatever foods and drinks are ingested into small molecules so as to nourish the body, provide energy, and repair cells. The digestive system is designed to provide the body with many vital amino acids, different forms of carbohydrates, fats, vitamins, and minerals. Without an adequate intake of these vital nutrients, history tells us that the human body would suffer. We need the energy from our food to perform, especially if we are attempting to work at an optimal level. The brain will then begin to relay messages to our cells to tell them what action to take and what hormones to make, causing the immune system to respond, positively or negatively, based on God's design for it. If there's a breakdown in any part of the digestive system, then "Houston, we have a problem!"

If you can recall in high school when you took biology, you learned the many different systems of the human body and how they all worked together. It's primarily responsible for our growth. The things we eat and drink have a strong effect not only on our bodies but also on our emotional and mental health.

Let's take a moment to imagine your dream car; let's say, a Mercedes Benz. Based on my research, a Mercedes Benz can cost between $40,000–$250,000. If we spent that kind of money on a car, most of us wouldn't dare put cheap gas, cheap oil, or any other cheap item in it. Why? Because we would naturally place a lot of value on that kind of car.

It's common knowledge that the manufacturers of the Mercedes Benz tell owners that substandard fuel could damage the car. However, we give our bodies substandard fuel consistently when we make it a habit to eat foods that have little to no nutritional value.

Stay with me! Let me point out that the Mercedes Benz can be traded in for another vehicle. It can be wrecked. It can lose its value. The list goes on and on.

Now imagine putting the wrong kind of gas into that Mercedes Benz, and the engine has a hard time processing that gas. Imagine also that the fumes from burning the wrong type of gas got trapped in the exhaust pipe, and those fumes were now backing up into the car where you were riding and driving. Is that a good visual?

The gas used to fuel the Mercedes is similar to the food used to fuel our bodies. The opening of gas tank is your mouth. Your esophagus is similar to the pipes that take the gas from your mouth to the engine. The stomach is the engine, where all the nutrients are absorbed. After the engine takes out what it needs for the well-being of the vehicle, the process of combustion, known as digestion in the human body, is completed by elimination of the waste products via the exhaust pipes. These exhaust pipes are your small and large intestines.

Many of our cars are designed to show a "check engine" light as soon as the system senses a problem. The body does the same thing when it gives off symptoms. If our pipes, or intestines, are clogged with some kind of debris, problems begin to arise. Releasing the waste products from our "vehicle" plays a major role in the vehicle running at optimal performance However, many of us ignore our bodies' "check engine" warnings.

How well do you think we would take care of our bodies if we valued them like we valued a Mercedes Benz? We can trade in a Mercedes Benz and get another car. But what can you trade this "earthly vehicle" in for? A heavenly one? Correct me if I'm wrong. No one is excited about trading in their "earthly body" for a "heavenly one!" I'm just saying!

STUDY GUIDE QUESTIONS

My Gift #1: What does Romans 12:1–2 mean to you?

_____

_____

_____

_____

_____

_____

My Gift #2: Share your thoughts on both of these statements:

She is wrong! I treated my earthly vehicle the same way I would treat a Mercedes Benz! Share three ways you took care of your expensive and very valuable body.

_____

_____

_____

_____

_____

She isn't wrong! I've disrespected my earthly vehicle! Share three ways that you wrecked your expensive and very valuable body.

_____

_____

_____

_____

_____

My Gift #3: List some of the "fuel" that you are putting in your body.

_____

_____

_____

_____

4. Is your "fuel" regular unleaded or premium unleaded?

_____

5. IF your body were a car, what kind of car would it be and how much would it cost?

_____

Chapter 2

The Diagnosis

In naturopathy and nutrition, the colon is where health and disease start. Even though there were bowel movements, something continually felt off. It was like my colon was still full and felt constricted. I continued to do my due diligence. Even though I was working on my doctorate in traditional naturopathy, I knew I needed someone else more experienced in this field than myself. I considered that my colon distress could possibly be linked to pinched nerves, and that it was wise to consult a chiropractor. Someone I trusted. I was beginning to feel desperate to resolve this matter as quickly as possible!

Initially, in an effort to resolve it myself, I started seeking God through prayer and personal study time to see what insight I could gain; but nothing came to mind. My philosophy: "When God isn't giving any insight, do what's natural until He provides directions." I also went to the health food store in Desoto to see if they could provide a different perspective. I was desperate not to fall into depression, or another debilitating gut issue. Because I was so desperate, I no longer cared about my image. My image was something that I had always held in very high regard. On this occasion, I freely shared all my personal business with the attendant at the store. I was willing to do whatever it took to get some help. I remember the lady giving me magnesium water, which provided a little relief, but it didn't immediately provide the relief I wanted. I instantly fell into a deep, dark state of despair right in the middle of the store in front of the attendant. As she watched my countenance change, she looked at me hopelessly. Her hopelessness mirrored exactly how I was feeling.

As I walked out of the health food store, the spirit of death confronted me in the parking lot. We were literally standing face to face. It was real! I felt it! I tried to rebuke it! I was alone and weak. All kinds of thoughts ran through my head. "Where is my family? Am I going to die by myself in this parking lot?" I was so overwhelmed with the thoughts of death and dying that I could literally feel the life leaving my body. I just knew that I was getting ready to die. While I stood in the parking lot, in tears, I cried out to the Lord. A subtle peace came over me in that moment. The Lord brought His peace and a part of me knew that everything would be alright. Simultaneously, another part of me didn't think His peace was enough.

My gut was still in distress! I just wanted the discomfort gone and I wanted it gone, like RIGHT NOW! "God, why can't you just snap your fingers and make this go away?" I knew that He was big enough! I wanted this test of faith to be over!

I left the parking lot that day feeling completely hopeless. Now, I know that it was another missed opportunity to get to know God. Another brush with death—not quite the way I wanted or expected this visit to the health food store to turn out.

After returning home, I felt depressed and went over to the dark-side for "tea and cookies." I did this for a couple of days. I didn't feel like praying.

Eventually, I came to the realization that I needed to be pressed into my Father like my life depended on it. I didn't feel like I had much of a choice. Desperate times call for desperate measures. I knew I had to take the next step. My body, my mind, and my emotions were demanding it. So I reached out to one of the professionals whom I had grown to trust, Dr. Silva. He was a chiropractor well versed in many of the natural therapies; and over the years, we had built a working relationship. We had similar philosophies on holistic modalities. I chose him to be one of my healthcare providers. I felt confident that he would help provide the answers I needed. After examining the lump on my back, he suggested that I go in for an x-ray at the local imaging center that day. I agreed so I went to get the x-ray of my spine to see what could possibly be going on. I knew from experience that a lump in the lower back was related to digestive issues.

When I arrived at the imaging center, they were advertising mammograms at the front desk. Every year or two, I had gotten a mammogram, so I knew that I was due. I figured that while I was at the imaging center I could knock out two birds with one stone. Little did I know that my "lump in the back" was just the beginning because, lo and behold, the technicians saw an image on the mammogram in the right breast. They immediately began to panic. They completely lost sight of my primary reason for being there. All my concerns about my back where overtaken by what they saw on the mammogram. They consulted with additional medical personnel who demanded that I act right away! That day to be exact! I asked them to allow me some time with my husband and my God before I launched into their suggestions. They became upset that I rejected their "right now" solution. Not that I was against doing anything medically. It just all happened so fast! I was in pure shock! I had learned from experience that God was holding me responsible for what I did or didn't do with my body, not the doctors.

In the midst of this negative situation, I had to speak some words of life to myself. I had memorized a Health and Wellness Decree given to me by one of my clients, Mrs. Valerie Johnson. When I got to my car, I immediately began to recite this decree out loud:

Health and Wellness Decree

Today, I present my body to you, oh Lord, for it is my reasonable servant. (Rom. 12:1) My body is the temple of the Holy Ghost, and I will not defile it. (2 Cor. 6:19–20)

I am accountable for the deeds done in body. (Rom. 14:12) My body is subjected to my spirit and my spirit is subjected to the Holy Spirit.

I will allow the Holy Spirit to be in charge of my will and my emotions that I might prosper and be in health. Father, you have given me intrinsic power over negative thoughts and actions, therefore I denounce low self-esteem.

I will lay aside every weight and sin that harasses me and I will run, with patience, the race that is set before me.

Because I wait on you Lord, my strength is renewed. I will mount up with wings of eagles. I will run and not be weary, I will walk and not faint. I declare my workout is my praise.

Therefore, I command my body to be energize. My body will respond with optimal proficiency. As I inhale positivity, I will exhale negativity.

I command blood flow to supply oxygen to all my organs, bones, joint, tendons, and ligaments with efficiency.

I declare that I am healed. I am more than a conqueror. Therefore, I will produce results of excellence, so in the name of Jesus, Father, receive my praise.

Because I was pursuing my doctorate in traditional naturopathy during this twilight adventure, I knew that if I didn't get the gut healthy, things wouldn't go well with the breast. Please don't get me wrong, I believe the medical community plays a vital role in our health. I also believe in and love being practical. One should use all the resources available to them and their family that will create the best quality of life. I believe practicality is one tool that I missed early in my Christian walk.

That being said, traditional naturopathy teaches that the gut is the foundation of the whole body. Sick gut, sick body. The breast had to take a "proverbial' second place to the immediate threat of system shutdown through the digestive path. Once again, hopelessness was upon me as I left the imaging center. I began to recognize a pattern of hopelessness in my thoughts. I "felt" like I had been in this negative space before. Somehow, this time was different. The hopelessness didn't overtake me like it done before. I attributed this to declaring the Health and Wellness Decree. However, I did ask the questions, "What in the world is going on, and where is God in all this? At that moment, I was more afraid of the gut issues than the now new threat of breast cancer. As I questioned "Lord Jesus, what the world, I heard a soft voice say, "Did you say you wanted to get to know me?" My immediate answer was, "Not like this!"

Study Guide Questions

My Gift #1: What part of the Health and Wellness Decree spoke to you immediately and profoundly?

_____

_____

_____

_____

_____

My Gift #2: Name a situation where it became obvious that you and God thought very differently on an issue or concern that you had.

_____

_____

_____

_____

My Gift #3: Take a moment and think about a relationship in which someone may have an unrealistic expectation of you. Use this example as a mirror to name three unrealistic expectations you have about your relationship with God Almighty.

_____

_____

_____

_____

_____

_____

_____

_____

CHAPTER 3

The Meltdown

This is a good place to talk about churchgoing and truly getting to know God on a personal level. I had this notion in my mind that God would answer my prayers based on how I thought the answer should be. I would say that this was one of the biggest "delusional truths" that had to be torn down in my mind. Answering my prayer in the way that I thought had become an idol instead of knowing God's will. Unfortunately, this is the focus for many churchgoers. We've made it about "answering our prayers" instead of seeking what God desires. If you really want to get to know God and His ways, let me encourage you to be open to the way that GOD DESIRES to answer your prayers! He isn't like humans. He has clearly stated in Isaiah 55: 8–13,

People Cannot Understand God

The LORD says, "My thoughts are not like yours.
Your ways are not like mine.
Just as the heavens are higher than the earth,
so my ways are higher than your ways,
and my thoughts are higher than your thoughts.
"Rain and snow fall from the sky
and don't return until they have watered the ground.
Then the ground causes the plants to sprout and grow,
and they produce seeds for the farmer and food for people to eat.
In the same way, my words leave my mouth,
and they don't come back without results.
My words make the things happen that I want to happen.
They succeed in doing what I send them to do.

"So you will go out from there with joy.
You will be led out in peace.
When you come to the mountains and hills, they will begin singing.
All the trees in the fields will clap their hands.
Large cypress trees will grow where there were thorn bushes.
Myrtle trees will grow where there were weeds.
All this will happen to make the Lord known,
to be a permanent reminder of his goodness and power."

As I continued to cry out to God for answers, I kept receiving emails from a place called Naturopathic Therapies. They were advertising specials on colonics. The first time I received an email, I deleted it, because I didn't know who it was from. The funny thing is that God was answering my prayer of deliverance, and I didn't even recognize it. I already had in my mind how God was going to answer me. Talk about unrealistic expectations!

The advertisement had to come two more times before the light bulb came on in my head. I had begun to get annoyed with this same email that kept coming after deleting it two times. The last time the email came the Lord said, "This is your answer." It certainly brought relief from hopelessness, despair, depression, and thoughts of death. This clinic was able to provide many tests that promoted natural health. Some of these tests verified the breast abnormalities from the imaging center. Little did I know that this would be the place where I was to do my internship for the doctorate of traditional naturopathy. It was an adventure and an opportunity to implement the principles and concepts that I had been learning and experiencing in this Naturopathic program. I worked feverishly for about 12–18 months to get my gut healthy. I was able to eat and digest my food without adverse effects. I had consistent bowel movements without the aid of laxatives, and my physical and mental health began to improve greatly. I started taking steps to put the breast as the primary focus. It was time. The thought of addressing another possible "engine failure" had me terrified of the possible outcome. It had to be done. This wasn't a time to stick my head in a hole or try to rebuke or confess it away. I had to be practical and spiritual simultaneously. My life was possibly at risk.

After healing the gut, I started the journey to address the breast. Many medical doctors refused to take me on as a patient because I was asking for other options. They literally thought that I had lost my mind to even ask for an alternative. I became very frustrated with the whole situation. They were interested in treating just the breast from a medical point of view;

however, as a student of traditional naturopathy, I was interested in holistic health. I also continued to seek a biblical perspective on how to address all my health concerns.

Since I had worked so hard to stabilize the digestive system, I felt compelled to protect it as much as possible. During this time, the Lord moved on the heart of one of my previous fitness clients, Mrs. Donna Gaines, who recommended that I talk to Dr. Jill Waggoner. Mrs. Gaines had shared many of my struggles about the medical disapproval of other physicians with Dr. Waggoner. Dr. Waggoner had also been informed that I was studying to become a traditional naturopath and was knowledgeable about some basic components of health. Because Donna and many of my other clients had spoken very highly of Dr. Waggoner, I decided to make an appointment. I didn't know that she, Dr. Waggoner, would eventually play a major role in where God was taking me concerning my health.

During my health crisis, none of the other doctors I saw were willing to hear what I had to say about my health concerns. Dr. Waggoner was the only one. God was ordering my steps to the people whom He wanted on my team for this journey.

As I met with Dr. Waggoner, the first order of the day was to get a biopsy. I did explain to Dr. Waggoner that my health was my responsibility and that I would be the primary decision maker in this journey, regardless of the outcome. She was in total agreement. The one thing I remember her saying to me was, "If I feel like you're being irrational about your health, it's my duty as a physician to tell you, but I'll still respect whatever decision you make." This was a statement that I had made to several of my clients when we were in training about their health. So, I knew that particular statement was God directly speaking to me about working with her on the next steps on my journey. This was one of many divine connections needed to get to the next step in my destination.

Based on how I had been learning the ways of God, my Father, I knew that I had to fortify my mind regarding all the possible outcomes of the biopsy. The Lord had been gracious to provide Dr. Waggoner as an open-minded medical doctor. I am very grateful for her. She is a woman of faith, full of God's power, and very open to other ways of obtaining health. She and I stood in prayer together as we scheduled the biopsy.

It was unnerving waiting on the results. So many thoughts ran through my mind. I tried so hard not to be afraid, but I decided I had to tell the Father the truth. I was petrified! Who wouldn't be?

That was the raw truth!

It's important to be honest with God. Many Christians feel that by voicing their fears to God, they're somehow displaying a lack of faith. Multiple times during this whole process, I was reminded by the Holy Spirit to keep it real with God as in John 4:23–24 where it says,

> "It's who you are and the way you live that counts before God. Your worship must engage your spirit in the pursuit of truth." That's the kind of people the Father is out looking for: those who are simply and honestly themselves before Him in their worship. God is sheer Being itself—Spirit. Those who worship him must do it out of their very being, their spirits, their true selves, in adoration.

I had to get "butt naked" spiritually before God. It was very ugly because my fleshly self lost all control! SheQuiQui, my ego, was on the rampage! "Why I am in this space?" I continually asked myself.

I later discovered that my emotional health was full of infection because I vomited words of sheer disrespect toward God, words of hatred, words fueled with anger and complete frustration. I didn't realize that this part of the infection had been festering in my heart and soul for a long time. I had been suppressing toxic, putrid, noxious, and venomous emotions and thoughts for years and didn't have any idea of what it was doing to my health mentally, physically, spiritually, relationally, and emotionally. I was completely shocked that a part of me felt this way toward God Almighty.

It was important to God that this "cancer of the soul" come to the light, just as the cancer of the body had. My emotional health so affected my physical well-being that my body was no longer willing, or capable of stuffing down any more poisonous thoughts or emotions. I would later learn that my emotions would be a direct link to my belief in my God and, ironically, the cancer. These cancers, of the soul and body, had to speak to get my attention. The disrespect had to stop in order to save my life. It was time to listen!

When cancer speaks, we listen! I was no different!

During this midnight hour of waiting for the biopsy results, I had to learn how to be still before the Lord. He called it listening. I called it boring! Talk about hard to be still! I started practicing yoga to learn how to be still.

Yoga and LEARNING HOW TO BE STILL was a major challenge. The environment of yoga caused me to pay attention to the thoughts that had been infiltrating my body, mind, and emotions. This was extremely disturbing to witness! It was like watching a horror movie without any popcorn and M&Ms. I began to understand why God admonished us about our thought life in 2 Corinthians 10:3–6 from *The Message*:

The world is unprincipled. It's dog-eat-dog out there! The world doesn't fight fair. But we don't live or fight our battles that way—never have and never will. The tools of our trade aren't for marketing or manipulation, but they are for demolishing that entire massively corrupt culture. We use our powerful God—tools for smashing warped philosophies, tearing down barriers erected against the truth of God, fitting every loose thought and emotion and impulse into the structure of life shaped by Christ. Our tools are ready at hand for clearing the ground of every obstruction and building lives of obedience into maturity.

I had to be taught to be still. Patiently, Mrs. Debi, my yoga instructor, did an excellent job of teaching me how to pull out my proverbial "yoga mat" and breathe in anticipation of the outcome.

My SheQuiQui (my ego, my human side) tried to play out several scenarios about the outcome of the biopsy. But, nothing could have prepared me for the variety of emotions that would flood my mind and soul.

That afternoon, I did all the breathing exercises that I could to protect the peace that I had worked so hard to obtain before returning to Dr. Waggoner's office for the results. I was determined to maintain a cool, calm, and collected disposition in the office in front of Dr. Waggoner.

She was as gracious as she could possibly be as she told me the life-shattering news. Stage 1 ductal carcinoma in situ. I sat still, pretending to be unshaken as shock assaulted my body while my mind refused to ingest the words. She asked me if I was okay and I assured her that I was, at that moment.

But when I got to the car, the wildfire of emotions came and washed over me like a tsunami wave. Disappointment, anger, frustration, unbelief, abandonment, and despair were expressed as poisonous words directed at God Almighty.

Yes, I did say directed at God Almighty!

"Why didn't He protect me? I served Him faithfully all these years and truly this isn't how I'm going out of here! How could God dishonor me in this fashion?"

Shortly following the fiery tsunami of emotions, I knew that I needed some help. I had enough presence of mind to call somebody. I called my mom first. I was speechless. She knew what the outcome of the biopsy had been because of my shear silence. All I could say was "Mom!" Nothing else would come out, but tears! She assured me that the Lord would see me through it all. She cried with me and began to pray for me. She calmed me down just by speaking God's words. Even now, while writing this, I feel those same emotions as though it were yesterday. I made it past the first wave of emotions as I ended the call with her.

By the time the second wave came, I was furious! All I could think about was all the sacrifices that I had made to serve God, and this was His way of rewarding me. Nothing made sense.

Nothing!

Indescribable darkness swept over my entire being. The second desperate call for help was to my dear friend, Nola Garrett. She had been my rock, my angel, my girlfriend for the past 20 years. She had embodied John 15:13, *"Greater love has no man than this, to lay down his life for a friend."* I am truly in debt to my God for her. How can I ever repay God for this woman who had been my angel in so many dark places? This time was no different. She assured me that she would be with me no matter what. That was a great comfort to me then, and continues to be a great comfort even now.

After talking to these two great women of God, I felt like I had the strength to face my husband with the news. I was able to talk to him without the devastation and fiery emotions in my voice. Of course, he had been holding his breath just as I had.

Before the diagnosis, I had underestimated the power of my emotional health. I believe many of us do. I began to learn that God designed our emotions to serve us as a sign post, not to master us. In this circumstance I had a decision to make: peace or fear? This entire situation was an opportunity for me to exercise my power to choose peace.

I chose fear!

Study Guide Questions

My Gift #1: After reading this section of the book, what words have you noticed coming out of your mouth?

_____

_____

_____

_____

My Gift #2: List three ways that your self-talk has affected your health and well-being:

_____

_____

_____

_____

My Gift #3:. Find an affirmation statement that speaks to you personally and confess it daily for 30 consecutive days. Track your changes in a journal.

_____

_____

_____

_____

CHAPTER 4

What? It's Not About ME?

As a student of traditional naturopathy, I knew all diseases began somewhere, mainly in the gut. I also knew the medical community played a part in the kingdom agenda and in my life, but I didn't know how.

This diagnosis caused me to press more into God for more answers. Not just any answers, but His specifically "Lord, you made this body. Where is this cancer coming from?"

God had promised me years ago, through a song He had given me when I was homeschooling my children, that His perspective was always available. During this trial, I sought God's perspective like the woman who searched for the lost coin in Luke 15:8–10. Still, it was hard for me to focus on His perspective because of my fear; because of my disappointment; because of my anger. I was devastated. On my most desperate and challenging days, when I was captivated by fear, I was able to take this song out of my arsenal in my fight to gain God's Perspective:

Don't Get Distracted

Don't get distracted; keep your mind on the Lord. You know it's easy for you to get bored.

Make your mind sit down and listen; bring your thoughts under God's submission.

When you focus, God will make it clear. And His voice you will hear.

He will give you the directions you need. All you have to do is believe.

Sing this song, sing this song; everybody come let's sing this song.

Let's sing this song, let's sing this song; everybody come let's sing!

Look to Jesus, he's the one who gives the power to overcome.

He called me out of darkness into the light; He put me on the path to do what's right.

Focus on Him, this will make you free; overcomers he made us to be.

The mind of Christ is yours for the asking; God's love for you is everlasting.

Sing this song, sing this song; everybody come let's sing this song.

Let's sing this song, let's sing this song; everybody come let's sing!"

Just focus on Him, just focus on Him, just focus on him, and it will be alright!

This song was also like a cloak of hope in my hands to overcome my thoughts of fear and despair. I found great comfort when I chose to sing it. As I sang the song, God began to unlock some of His secrets on health. The more I used this song as a weapon, the more God began to give me insight into why He talked so much about praise and worship.

Words are powerful! Words have creative power, whether positive or negative.

He made it clear to me that many of my negative words and emotions had a detrimental effect on my health. My negative self-talk had been instrumental in many of my health challenges. I began to understand why He admonished us in 1 Thessalonians 5:18 to *give thanks in everything, for this is the will of God concerning us.* Words have a powerful effect on cellular health. Our body cells don't just absorb nutritional food and drink, they absorb words as well. God has spoken many times throughout Scriptures on the tongue and what comes out of our mouths. God explained to me in detail that I had been feeding my body, mind, and cells words of poison. I like the way *The Message* explains James 3: 3–10 about the power of the mouth and words.

A bit in the mouth of a horse controls the whole horse. A small rudder on a huge ship in the hands of a skilled captain sets a course in the face of the strongest winds. A word out of your mouth may seem of no account, but it can accomplish nearly anything—or destroy it! It only takes a spark, remember, to set off a forest fire. A careless or wrongly placed word out of your mouth can do that. By our speech we can ruin the world, turn harmony to chaos, throw mud on a reputation, send the whole world up in smoke and go up in smoke with it, smoke right from the pit of hell. This is scary: You can tame a tiger, but you can't tame a tongue—it's never been done. The tongue runs wild, a wanton killer. With our tongues we bless God our Father; with the same tongues we curse the very men and women he made in his image. Curses and blessings out of the same mouth!

During my journey of addressing the breast cancer, I had so many mixed emotions about praying. I won't lie. There were some days when I desperately wanted to hear His Perspective. I wanted the Lord to talk to me and I was willing to listen. On the other days, I didn't want to talk to Him. And you could forget about wanting to listen. I didn't know what to expect from Him.

I got to a point where I could began asking questions of the Lord again. I had many questions. I wanted to understand. A part of me still had a great desire to know God, while another part of me sulked over the idea of this great trial.

My dear friend and sister, Nola, was truly an angel while I was in this dark place. She prayed for me. She prayed with me. She prayed at me. She prayed, prayed, prayed! She prayed me out of the dungeon when there was no flashlight! She kept it real with me. She would tell me that she was afraid for me, but she kept telling me that God was going to show up. It was comforting to know that I wasn't alone in my fears.

During the dark times, there was nothing humbling about my attitude toward God at all. I had an attitude of entitlement. I felt like God owed me. I had based my Christian life on Psalms 37:4 where it says that *if I delighted myself in the Lord, He would give me the desires of my heart.* I had taken Psalms 37:4 to mean that if I were a good girl for the kingdom of God, He would give me **whatever I wanted**!

When I finally recognized that the principle of obedience wasn't a recipe for God giving me what I wanted, it was life changing. I eventually began to understand that it was a recipe from God to give me the best life that He has chosen for me. Previous to this, in my mind, I had lived a life of obedience to the hard things that I believed God had called me to do. Things like: staying married; homeschooling; not working a full-time job outside of the home; and giving the finances over to my husband, although I had a degree in Business Administration Accounting. I could go on and on. I think you get the picture!

Well, for me, when I got on the other side of Psalms 37:4, I didn't expect a breast cancer diagnosis. I had to deal with my disappointment, frustration, and anger. SheQuiQui (my ego) was acting like a worldly, carnal, arrogant, nonbeliever. I was extremely angry and disappointed that God had allowed me to be in this head space. "How could He let me fall into this darkness after all I've done for Him?"

Believe it or not, there was a time during this journey when I turned my back on God. I no longer wanted to serve the Lord, if this was the way He was going to treat me.

Yet He pursued me and loved on me anyway.

I remember the Lord distinctly telling me that He wasn't intimidated by my attitude. He continued to talk to me like a Father to a rebellious and immature child. I was truly acting like a 2-year-old. I was in a full-fledged tantrum. Can you tell that maybe I was thinking that this was all about me? I didn't stop for one moment to consider that, maybe, this cancer diagnosis could be God's answer to many prayers I had prayed to reach the lost. During this process, God spoke to me daily, explaining His purpose in the midst of this problem.

Oh, I can hear your thoughts! *How dare she say that God allowed this! Doesn't she know that it was Satan?*

Yes, it was Satan showing forth through my destructive, negative attitudes! The Lord made me aware that I had opened the door to Satan, and invited him in for proverbial tea and cookies!

The Lord would also impart to me the importance of knowing those areas that weren't fully submitted to him, but were still dedicated to living life in love with sin, self, and Satan.

Come on saints! We have to take some personal responsibility for our actions and behaviors so that we can understand the connection to our health and well-being. We blame so much of our immature behaviors on Satan and others; but when are we going to start looking at what we need to do to respect God the way He wants to be respected? I had never asked God how He wanted to be respected, because I never realized that He had a way that He wanted to be respected. I assumed I already knew how He wanted to be respected. That was my error!

Even after I made the decision to return to God, it was difficult to listen to Him. As these daily conversations with God continued to flood my mind, I resumed listening to what was being said. One profound idea that impacted me during this time was when I heard, "You say you want to be used by Me, but you have decided on how this is to be done. I am the author and the finisher of your faith, so I get to decide what I will use for my kingdom." These kind of thoughts kept coming to my mind. One day, as I was walking across the threshold at Sprouts, I suddenly heard these thoughts flood my mind: "There are so many struggling with cancer. So many people hurting. The fields are ripe for the picking, but the laborers are few. I need you to be willing to go into the darkness, where people are hurting, take them hope, and bring them out of darkness." At this time, my heart began to soften. I didn't know if I was up for the challenge. God was providing His perspective on the problem, and how He wanted to use it for His purpose. This was one of my flashlights in the darkness.

The kingdom of God has given us a lot of power to change our lives, and also to be instrumental in changing the lives of others. Unfortunately, I was ignorant on how to access this power, even though I was going to church. I knew something was lacking in my Christian walk. I would read Scriptures and compare it to my life and wonder, "God, what I am missing?" I knew there had to be more to life than what I was experiencing. We play a part in this scenario of broken lives, especially our own. This "health opportunity" was a major shift in my belief system. It required that I think differently on my relationship with God. I did learn that God's definitions and my definitions of biblical principles were vastly different. They were worlds apart. Haven't you heard this Scripture said, or perhaps even quoted it for yourself?

"For my thoughts are not your thoughts, neither are your ways my ways, said the Lord? For as the heavens are higher than the earth, so are my ways higher than your ways, and my thoughts than your thoughts" (Isa. 55:8–10).

If you are seeking God for His opinions and perspective on your life, stand ready for Him to answer you the way He knows is best for you and your circumstances. It does say in Jeremiah 29: 11 that He knows the plans He has for us. Sometimes this can be easy to say, but tough to do. Do we really want to trust Him if it means we must give up the control of our lives? What if He is asking us to accept and embrace the process that He has chosen of you getting His answers, especially if it doesn't look like the way you want it to?

As you take the time to pray, learn to listen to what God has to say. Ask God to help you accept His answers and the way He chooses to answer you. Is your relationship with God really about doing what He desires, or is it about you getting everything that you want based on your definition of life? If He is calling you to let Him be in control, it has got to be on his terms, not yours!

STUDY GUIDE QUESTIONS

My Gift #1: Name one area of your life where God's way of doing things is completely different than your way of doing things.

_____

_____

_____

_____

My Gift #2: Has your Christian walk been mostly about what you want or what God wants?

_____

My Gift #3: Have you prayed to be a witness for the kingdom of God? Write one way that you have asked God to use you.

_____

_____

_____

_____

_____

_____

My Gift #4: Did you consider the price that you might have pay? Usually in order to be effective in ministry, it's important that you go through the journey first. What journey has God called you on in order to take hope to the hopeless?

_____

_____

_____

_____

_____

My Gift #5: What thoughts, attitudes, and emotions surfaced as you read James 3:3–10?

_____

_____

_____

_____

_____

_____

CHAPTER 5

A Search for a Guarantee

After my biopsy results came back, Dr. Waggoner recommended I see an oncologist. My nerves were shot as I was on my way to my first appointment.

When I arrived, this oncologist looked to be in her late 20s to early 30s. That was my first warning sign. My nerves escalated ten times over, and my confidence in her abilities dropped to an all-time low.

I usually don't tell medical doctors right up front what I do as a profession. I like to see where their ideologies rest before I disclose such controversial information. Traditional naturopaths and medical doctors come from completely different philosophies.

In most Western societies, the majority of people give the responsibility of their health to doctors. I had been one of those people, but God had begun to explain to me how He wanted me to respect Him in the area of overall health. He explained the kind of respect that He desires in Romans 12:1–2 where He tells us:

Brothers and sisters, God has shown you his mercy. So I am asking you to offer up your bodies to him while you are still alive. Your bodies are a holy sacrifice that is pleasing to God. When you offer your bodies to God, you are worshiping him in the right way. Don't live the way this world lives. Let your way of thinking be completely changed. Then you will be able to test what God wants for you. And you will agree that what he wants is right. His plan is good and pleasing and perfect.

He had called me into accountability to Him and His purposes with regard to my body, mind, and emotions.

The word *cancer* will cause anyone to abandon their health responsibility by automatically taking the path of least resistance. I get it.

When I heard the "C" word, I just wanted somebody to make it go away, or tell me that a mistake had been made on the biopsy. Let me tell you, even though I had education about health from a natural perspective, I was just as scared as the average person. I just wanted the situation resolved, as quickly as possible. I prayed during the whole visit with this oncologist. I kept asking God, "Where are you in this? You said you are always at work around me. I can't see you!"

She was in the room for only 2 minutes before she offered up what seemed like a script: Lumpectomy with radiation, or double mastectomy with reconstruction.

Her words and how she talked to me made me feel like I was just another number. She displayed no compassion at all. She didn't ask me one personal question, and had the audacity to get upset when I told her that I would have to discuss her suggestions with my husband first.

I quickly decided that she wasn't the person to be on my team for the breast cancer journey. Apparently, she didn't get the memo that my health was my decision. I informed her that I decided to get a second opinion. As a result of my decision, she informed the insurance company that I wasn't compliant with her recommendations. I wasn't opposed to her recommendations. I just knew she didn't have my best interests in mind. I wanted someone who was willing to listen to the questions and concerns I had about this drastically life-changing event.

As I hadn't received any insight from God on the matter, I went to get a second opinion. During this whole process, one of my clients had suggested a natural option. She had begun to send me information about a place called Optimum Health Institute (OHI). At the time, I was still having significant issues wrapping my mind around this diagnosis. Completely understandable, right?

The second oncologist was definitely more attentive, more compassionate. She treated me like I mattered. The visit was actually about 40 minutes long. She allowed me to ask questions. She offered different solutions, none of which were natural. She was in no rush to do surgery, but surgery was certainly part of the solutions she offered. She did a great job of explaining the procedure, as well as her rationalization behind it.

As we discussed several options, the one question that completely turned the tables and seem to have created the environment for God to show up was this: "I've spent the last year to eighteen months working to get my digestive system working properly, so I could address my breast. Could you tell me how this surgery will affect my digestive system?" Her reply was very compassionate, as she said with a heavy heart, "Ma'am, we don't care anything about your digestive system; all we care about is the removal of the cancer."

Right after the doctor said those words, I heard a voice in my head say, "You're looking for someone to guarantee that whatever decision you make will lead to healing and not take your life. No one can offer that, but Me."

That thought sent me into a tizzy. As I walked out of the doctor's office and stood on the sidewalk, looking for my vehicle, I heard myself responding back, "Of course, I'm looking for a guarantee!"

My fears were telling me that I needed to make a decision soon, but I wasn't quite ready to make one yet. I had not gathered all the information I needed to make a sound decision, and I still hadn't gotten any specific directions from Heaven. At this time, I decided to take my client's advice to visit the OHI center to see what they had to offer.

Study Guide Questions

My Gift #1: Name one decision that you're contemplating that has the potential to drastically change your life.

_____

   A. Write the pros:

_____

_____

_____

_____

   B. Write the cons:

_____

_____

_____

_____

If the pros outweigh the cons, it's probably the best decision for you, not just in health, but on any issue of life.

If the cons outweigh the pros, it's probably not the best decision for you.

My Gift #2: Decision are one of our power sources. Some decisions you can recover from. Some decisions will cost you your life. Have you ever viewed your decisions as your source of power?

_____

_____

_____

My Gift #3: Reflect on your past decisions. Which ones brought life to you and your family? Which ones didn't?

Be careful how you make decisions.

_____

_____

_____

_____

_____

_____

CHAPTER 6

Quality of Life

I continued to seek the Lord on what directions I needed to take concerning the cancer diagnosis. My faith level was in seed form. It had absolutely no roots. Yet. It had only been planted into my human reasoning for a short while. So much of my human reasoning was at the forefront of my mind. This just didn't make sense to me.

The Lord had really pushed me to a place I had never ever considered going or being in. I had never been in this kind of head space before, and I didn't know of anyone who had traveled a holistic pathway with regard to any kind of cancer. God had called me to a place where I didn't have anyone as a role model or mentor to turn to. In my mind, God had asked for this kind of sacrificial obedience before when He asked for me to give up a career and work at home; buy a car for someone who was a nonrelative; and, most of all, surrender the family finances to my husband. At the time, all of these "faith" steps brought about a tremendous amount of fear. This new walk of trusting God, to use natural therapies on this breast cancer journey, brought a fear I had hoped I would never have to experience again. However, even with trepidation, I took one baby step at a time!

My husband and I decided to visit the Optimum Health Institute in Austin, Texas. I had read many powerful testimonies on their website, and those testimonies gave me hope. Knowing all of the viable options made it easier to make informed decisions about my health. Little did I know that the Lord would meet me on the initial visit with the first installation of divine directions.

It took us about 3–4 hours to get to the beautiful facilities of OHI. It was tucked away from the mainstream in the middle of nowhere. There was nothing convenient within miles. It was literally surrounded by farm houses and land. It was like they were purposeful in being hidden. It would seem outlandish for a miracle designed by God to be in such a location.

Isn't that just like our Lord? Many times, He is in places that we wouldn't think, or desire, to look. However, if we want God's plan for our lives, we have to be willing to do it on His terms.

After we met all the staff, we began the tour. As the facilitator of the orientation started the tour, I noticed a Caucasian lady, who looked to be in her mid to late 40s, walking around in the hallways. She was walking very slowly, and appeared to be still struggling with some health issues. At first glance, I assumed she was battling cancer. Just a guess. It didn't look like she had any eyebrows, eyelashes, and she wore a head bonnet. She was extremely pale and fragile. As the tour came to an end, the Institute provided dinner. It was all raw food! Nothing was cooked or processed! Even though I was very familiar with clean eating, this kind of nutrition was on a whole other level! This was "holistic" nutrition!

Well, the lady I noticed earlier was named Julie. She sat at our table and she began to share her story with everyone seated there. It was like she was talking specifically to me. I started to wonder if she had heard my prayers to God.

Julie began to tell the story of how she had encountered cancer three times, each five years apart. She began to tell us about each encounter. In the first encounter, she went to the Cancer Treatment Centers of America where she had a lumpectomy, and a healing nutritional protocol was incorporated into her diet. She then told us that while she was at the center, she did as the team of doctors had instructed. However, unfortunately, when she returned home, she fell back into her old lifestyle patterns. She shared with us that she went back home, and instead of putting her health needs first, she continued to put the needs of her family first. Her nutrition went back to foods that were convenient for her family.

Boy, it was like I was looking in a mirror at myself when she said that. For years, I had thought that putting the needs of my family first was the Christian thing to do. To be perfectly honest, in my mind, I looked for opportunities to deny myself because I had presumed that it was a way to honor God. Wait a minute! Well, wasn't that what Luke 9:23 was talking about when it says to deny yourself and take up your cross and follow Christ?

For many years I had been feeling like something in my faith walk was missing, but I just didn't know what it was. I had been asking God to show me truth as He saw truth; and lo and behold, another Scripture that I had lived my life by was now being challenged by this woman's journey with cancer.

Julie continued to tell us about how the cancer revisited her 5 years later, and how it had metastasized to her lungs. For her second confrontation with cancer, Julie chose conventional methods as her weapons of choice. A double mastectomy with radiation and chemotherapy. That left her weak and vulnerable to many types of infections. But, even after experiencing the drastic measures to save her life, Julie told us that she still didn't change her lifestyle. Life went on as usual, still serving others, while serving herself last or not at all.

By this time, I was wondering where in the world God was in Julie's life if cancer came back for a second time. I had just graduated as a doctor of traditional naturopathy, and was still wet behind the ears as I analyzed this lady's testimony from a scientific, and spiritual, point of view. It was obvious that education doesn't equal experience. Something just wasn't adding up.

It was all just blowing my mind! Was all of this, my years of health crises one after another, about change? It sounded too simple; but obviously, she hadn't read the memo from heaven!

When the cancer showed up again 5 years later for the third time, it had spread to her brain. The doctors told her family that they had done all that they knew to do, and they eventually sent her home with hospice.

My husband and I were gripping our hands under the table, as though we didn't anticipate a hopeful ending to her story. I was certainly waiting for her to tell me that God had done something. I really needed hope. I wasn't quite ready to leave this world yet. I felt I had too many dreams left inside of me that needed to be shown to myself and the world.

Julie began to conclude her story by telling us that she was an active Christian in her church. She, like most of us, went to church on Wednesday for Bible study, Sunday morning Sunday school, intercessory prayer, and church service. "Where was the power of God?" I asked her where God was in all of this. Her initial reply was that she had lost all hope. She couldn't see Him, couldn't feel His presence, or trace His steps. Yet in her darkest moment, when she felt like all hope was lost, God had sent her a message of hope. I called this a place of surrender. It feels like crap! No one is preaching that kind of surrender!

Yet it's easy to get up and go to church on Sunday morning, and sing loud about how we surrender. I must say, many of my health challenges had begun to teach me not to sing about what I could do for God. Rather, they taught me to proclaim who God was and is. His faithfulness toward us. His unfailing love and how He deserves all the praise, glory, and honor.

This was another opportunity for me to see how important it was to learn how to listen to the words I was speaking in prayer and in song. What I call surrender and what God calls surrender are two totally different pictures.

Just when she thought that there was nothing anyone else could do for her, God sent a messenger from her church to let her know that He was and still is faithful! Someone from Julie's church told her about the miracles that were happening at OHI. Julie also explained that she and her family didn't have the financial means for her to go to OHI; but the lady from her church volunteered to pay for her to go to OHI for a week. Just the first week at OHI is $1,500! My mind was blown! This was the kind of hope I needed.

She wasn't finished, much to my surprise. I asked her how long she had been in the program and again her answer filled my husband and me full of hope. She had been in the holistic program for only one full week, seven consecutive days! I couldn't believe it. The woman, whom I initially viewed as frail and weak, was actually a walking miracle!

Her description of her initial arrival at OHI read like this: death was imminent, her skin color was gray. She wasn't able to walk on her own, so she was brought into the facility in a wheelchair. She had needed assistance going to the bathroom (someone else her to wipe her behind). She couldn't feed herself, and quality of life didn't exist for her. She was discouraged in her faith, but our God came through and gave her the hope that only He could give!

What in the world just took place? Eppie and I looked at each other with utter amazement, with hearts full of hope, and faces shining like God had just smiled on us! He and I embraced like we knew we had found our answer.

Julie welcomed questions from all who sat at the table. Her words would serve as the perspective that I had been seeking God for. Julie said, "The staff has not promised that this program would heal me or save my life, so I accept that the cancer may take my life. But what they did promise was this program would give me the best quality of life with whatever days I had left!" She declared the week that she had been at OHI had literally given her a quality of life that she had not known for a while. She considered wiping her own behind, feeding herself, and walking the halls, even though slow, as "quality of life" Many of the things she mentioned as quality of life, I knew I had been taking them for granted. Gratitude flowed out of her pores!

She displayed a demeanor that spoke to the truth that every day is a gift, so we must learn to live in the present. Easy to say, hard to practice. She really believed that it would be up to God to determine her last days. She didn't seem to be worried about dying because He has declared that we belong to him and that He is the author and the finisher of our faith! God has spoken of the life that He has come to give us: *"The thief comes only in order to steal and kill and destroy. I came that they may have and enjoy life, and have it in abundance [to the full, till it overflows]."* John 10:10 AMP.

I knew that God was challenging me to look at this diagnosis as an opportunity to experience quality of life, and not necessarily a demand for healing, or even to save my life. Of course, I was demanding the healing and not Him!

Laughing out Loud!

Could I accept that God would allow this diagnosis to be my exit from this world? If He's really God, does he have the power over life and death? Was this really how my life was going to end? This experience caused me to examine my faith in God.

If I'm honest with myself, that's really what this was all about. It's easy to praise God and trust God when things are going my way. That was a hard pill to swallow, but it provoked some thought and certainly prayer. I wasn't ready to die, but Julie taught me that I needed to hear what God had to say about my life, and not what I wanted Him to say.

Finally, I felt like I had some of God's directions for my life concerning the breast cancer. Even though the fear of dying had not left my thoughts, my husband and I decided that OHI and quality of life was the road that I would choose to take.

Part of me was excited about OHI because I felt like I had some directions, but another part of me was afraid because I didn't know what to expect.

On the drive to OHI for my first week, my hubby and I talked about getting certain affairs in order. It was sobering, but necessary.

Study Guide Questions

My Gift #1: What is your greatest takeaway from Julie's story?

_____

_____

_____

_____

_____

My Gift #2: Instead of demanding that God do things your way, are you willing to ask Him what He wants in whatever your challenge is today?

_____

_____

My Gift #3: What prayer do you see God answering in the midst of one of your greatest challenge?

_____

_____

_____

_____

My Gift #4: I know that this subject is not one that most people like to talk about, but do you have your affairs in order (Burial, Wills, Power of Attorney, etc.)

_____

CHAPTER 7

God's Perspective on the Root

Previous to the cancer diagnosis, my husband and I had a tough time getting on the same page with at least 50% of the issues concerning our marriage and family. A lot of my despairing emotions stemmed from our constant fighting over finances. Even though we were both Christians, it seemed like we constantly had "intense fellowship" over something.

I was so ready to leave my husband. We had been married for over 25 years, and I just knew that I had missed something about this thing called "marriage covenant." To me, it was more like a marriage war! It was martial, not marital. Many times, when I was convinced that our marriage was over and that I was leaving, my faith in God would intervene in a very profound way. Inevitably, I would stay. I stayed, not because I cared anymore, but because I KNEW that God was telling me to stay. I even told my husband the only reason that I had stayed in this marriage was because of my faith in the Lord Jesus Christ. Once again, just keeping it real.

After the diagnosis, it was amazing to see how my husband and I worked so well together under the threat of cancer. It took my breath away! What is it about life's difficulties that has the power to drive a husband and wife together to work on a common goal? A very specific goal.

This had not been the usual pattern in the past. It's like he automatically knew his part and I knew my part for this adventure. This was one of the first times in our marriage that I felt like my husband was protecting me. I'm not trying to make him look bad. I'm simply stating my perspective! That was my experience, and I did express those feelings of "not being protected" by him for many years.

Believe it or not, God allowed me to see that I had been in the way of my husband being the leader in our family. He desired to be the leader, but I was so afraid to let him lead. I was afraid of his leadership style. The image of what I thought was supposed to be a "strong Black woman" took a blow! I was able to see that it took a situation of this magnitude to get me to humble myself so that my husband could stand up and walk in his rightful God-given position.

Once I decided to go to OHI, my husband called a family meeting to get our adult children to help fund my decision for a holistic approach to the diagnosis. Our finances weren't in order, and he (we) knew that it would take a family effort for me to go to OHI.

The first week at OHI was going to cost us about $2,000 and about $1,200 for each additional week I decided to stay. Because of our lack of agreement on the finances in the past, we didn't have $2,000 saved up. Embarrassing, but true. It was because of the past mismanagement of income, a heavy debt load, a difference of opinion on money, and my not working a full-time job.

Before my diagnosis, the husband I knew would not have shared that with his adult children for fear of their image of him being destroyed. My husband was and still is a very giving man, almost to a fault. He had done a great job painting the kind of image that he wanted his children to view him in, especially his six boys! Even though it was humbling, my husband led the way in sharing with our children on how he had mismanaged the finances, and how we could accomplish this goal by pooling our monies together as a family. I stood in shock!

Before this "opportunity," my husband and I didn't pray together, seek God for His perspective on our issues, eat dinner together as a family, or consistently work on the finances. The one thing that we did do was go to church and have intense fellowship together. However, once we came to a decision, my husband took on the leadership role. Which meant that I had to get somewhere and sit down!

My husband was and still is the ultimate optimist, and I'm still a realist. In the past, those two perspectives didn't work well together. This diagnosis was a time that we drew closer to each other and to the Lord as a unit and to God's perspective.

This situation brought the best out in us. How was this possible? It was like we flourished well under the duress.

Crazy!

At this point, it did cross my mind that I was already starting to benefit from this diagnosis. Another prayer answered? Many years I had spent praying for us to work together, but certainly I didn't expect this!

We started praying together on a regular basis, without me prodding him. Discussing the finances was very intentional and great progress was made with the funds that we had available. He was willing to do whatever he needed to do, plus more, to make this life-changing event work to our advantage. He made sure the household chores were done and insisted on me resting as much as possible. Arguments between us came to a screeching halt! We were very careful about how we talked to each other. He made me feel like I was his number one priority because, in the past, I had told him that he was cheating on me with his job. Watching him in action was powerful. I was perplexed as to why it took something like this to bring us together. He became the physical representation of Christ. We were "becoming one" as stated in Ephesians 5:29–31

No man hates himself. He takes care of his own body. That is the way Christ does. He cares for His body which is the church. We are all a part of His body, the church. For this reason, a man must leave his father and mother when he gets married and be joined to his wife. The two become one.

We started this program as ONE. That alone is a miracle in itself.

On day one, an explanation was provided before each aspect of the holistic program at Optimum Health. Their program was very thorough when it came to health and wellness. It covered spirit, soul, body, emotions, social life, relationships, thoughts, exercise, nutrition, and the big "S" word, stress! They had scientific classes, spiritual classes, and classes that helped to balance out the physical body. All the food that was provided was raw and therapeutic for wholeness.

The nutritional protocol was also explained for people diagnosed with cancer. It was a very strict green juice regimen. Even though juicing was a major part of the program, I soon found out that wheatgrass would take the show.

They had the benefits of wheatgrass posted throughout the facilities. It was like green blood. As a student of naturopathy, I had not given much thought to wheatgrass as such a powerful agent of healing. It would prove to be one of God's many superfoods in the upcoming days. After the introduction to the nutritional program, a group devotional was encouraged. Those devotionals seemed like they were straight from the mouth of God, specifically orchestrated for the people who were there at that moment. I drew very close to the people on staff, as well as those who were confronting their own "health opportunities."

While there, the staff encouraged light exercise, as well as plenty of good, old fashioned, clean water! They had a selection of classes to choose from based on individual health concerns. After taking a class, one of the things I found tantalizing was their perspective on cancer. They kept referring to it as a "health opportunity." It really made a difference on how I began to look at this frightening challenging that seem to threaten my life. I would soon view it from a completely different perspective that was life changing.

During my time at OHI I began to learn that in Ephesians 2:5–10 that God's perspective was always available to me because of what Christ had done.

We were dead because of our failures, but he made us alive together with Christ. (It is God's kindness that saved you.) God has brought us back to life together with Christ Jesus and has given us a position in heaven with him. He did this through Christ Jesus out of his generosity to us in order to show his extremely rich kindness in the world to come. God saved you through faith as an act of kindness. You had nothing to do with it. Being saved is a gift from God. It's not the result of anything you've done, so no one can brag about it. God has made us what we are. He has created us in Christ Jesus to live lives filled with good works that he has prepared for us to do. God's Word Translation.

Change your perspective, change your life.

STUDY GUIDE QUESTIONS

My Gift #1:. Name one "health opportunity" that you want to gain God's Perspective on.

_____

My Gift #2: Name three perspectives of yours that you need to change.

_____

_____

_____

My Gift #3: Are you ready and willing to change them?

_____

My Gift #4:. Time for an Action Plan. Are you ready to change?

_____

5. Time for SMART Goals for self-care—
   Specific—Be specific.
   Measurable—Map it out.
   Achievable—Make the goal attainable.
   Relevant—Make it impact your life and health.
   Time-based—Set a realistic time in which you would like to
   see it accomplished.

_____

_____

_____

_____

_____

_____

_____

_____

_____

_____

_____

_____

_____

_____

Take the time to develop your new self-care habits by:

- Finding an accountability partner, someone you trust, someone who will help pull you to your greatness, someone who is an example of your desired destination.

- Being consistent one step at a time; take baby steps in establishing new habits.

- Being patient with yourself in developing these new habits.

CHAPTER 8

You Created It; You Can Uncreate It

As I began to get involved in the classes, view the documentaries, and the movies, that provided valuable information on how the body, mind, emotions, and thoughts worked, the Lord downloaded an idea to my unprepared mind. The information had begun to create an environment, in my mind, for God to download his thoughts in my heart where I could understand and make changes willingly. "You have created this," I clearly heard Him say to me. "If you created it, you can uncreate it."

This statement was so far "outside the box" thinking that it completely dumbfounded me. What could God possibly mean that I created it? The Scriptures began to make sense where God had spoken of our thought life, and how he admonished us against complaining;

> *Casting down imaginations, and every high thing that exalts itself against the knowledge of God, and bringing into captivity every thought to the obedience of Christ." (2 Cor. 10:5 KJV)*

> *In everything give thanks: for this is the will of God in Christ Jesus concerning you. (1 Thess. 5:18 KJV)*

These Scriptures, among many others, began to illuminate my mind. The thoughts, behaviors, and decisions that were based on sin, self, Satan, and the world's system of thinking, that I had so consistently and intensely dwelled on over the years, and that I talked about continually had created sickness and disease in my body. I began to understand Scriptures like:

For they that are after the flesh do mind the things of the flesh; but they that are after the Spirit the things of the Spirit. For to be carnally minded is death; but to be spiritually minded is life and peace. Because the carnal mind is enmity against God: for it is not subject to the law of God, neither indeed can be. (Rom. 8:5–7 KJV).

The lightbulb had been turned on. There was no going back to life as I had known it.

The absolutely fascinating thing that stood out in all of this download from God was that I felt hopeful instead of the hopelessness that I had come to OHI with. Think about that. What thoughts, behaviors, attitudes, or lifestyle habits have you been feeding that created your dilemmas? "If you created it, you have power to uncreate it!" That's a lot of power. Don't you think?

Study Guide Questions

My Gift #1: As Christians, we are great at praying and telling God what we want and need. However, in order to get to know the Lord on His terms, we must learn how to listen to what He has to say to us through our thoughts, emotions, and physical bodies. Many of us are "bleeding out" in some area that's hidden away from the human eye, but it's showing up in our physical bodies. Listen to the warning signs. It's very important to learn how to be still and listen to your own needs. The Lord cares for all of you.

_____

_____

_____

_____

_____

_____

_____

Meditation is the first component on which to build your health.

My Gift #2: Start by taking 5 minutes to just sit and listen to your thoughts, emotions, and physical sensations in your body without judgment. Pay attention to what you are seeing, hearing, and feeling. Journal about it. Take steps to bring care to these areas of concern. Benefits of meditation: increases self-awareness, teaches you how to listen to your internal needs, helps to reduce stress, promotes self-care, and helps the body to repair.

_____

_____

_____

_____

_____

My Gift #3: Typically, when we think about nutrition, we think only of food. However, in the world of traditional naturopathy, nutrition is about not only the foods we eat but also the thoughts/words we feast on, the words we drink in, the emotions that consume us, and the relationships that we feed on. Several studies have verified that thoughts/words, emotions, and relationships all have a profound effect on our health. Take some time to examine how you have been "feeding."

_____

_____

_____

_____

_____

_____

_____

_____

CHAPTER 9

My Injury

For years, I had been so displeased with my life in so many areas as a Christian. I had chosen to put my career on hold to raise my children for the kingdom of God, and because of it, I had built my belief system to my Savior based on Psalms 37:4 (KJV): *"Delight thyself also in the Lord, and he shall give thee the desires of thine heart."* I had my own definition of what that Scripture meant for me. I held onto it for many years, especially when things got tough and I thought about how I should have put career first, family second.

My expectation stemmed from the "good girl" complex. You know what that is, right? It is the mindset that if I do what God says, then He will give me what I want. I would tell myself "I just have to be a good girl no matter what! It will pay off."

Paradoxically, I was also praying that God would give me a heart that desired truth. I was soon to find out that the two antithetical philosophies: give me what I want and give me a heart of truth, didn't fit into the same fish bowl. Once again, I had no idea of what I'm asking for and the Lord was teaching me that He didn't see things the way I did. That prayer for truth was becoming a reality, but I was still holding onto the "good girl" mindset.

While at OHI, I began to discover the root cause for this mindset as well as other negative thoughts and emotions. As things began to happen that brought erroneous teaching and beliefs out in the open, God began to uproot that Scripture that I had built my goals and dreams on. He recalled to my mind that I had pray for truth. Then, He came in like a wrecking ball! I was reminded of the Scripture in Malachi 3:1–5 (NLV):

See, I am going to send one with news, and he will make the way ready before me. Then all at once the Lord you are looking for will come to His house. The one with the news of the agreement, whom you desire, is coming," says the Lord of All. "But who can live through the day of His coming? Who can stand when He shows Himself? For He is like a fire for making gold pure, and like a strong cleaner. He will sit as one who melts silver and makes it pure. He will make the sons of Levi pure. He will make them pure like gold and silver, so that they may bring the right gifts to the Lord. Then the gifts of Judah and Jerusalem will be pleasing to the Lord, as they were in the past. Then I will come to judge you. I will be quick to speak against those who use witchcraft, and those who do sex sins, and those who make false promises. I will speak against those who do not pay a man what he has earned, and who make it hard for the woman whose husband has died and for children who have no parents. And I will speak against those who turn away the stranger and do not fear me," says the Lord of All.

Now that I was experiencing this in my soul, it was like an implosion of an old building. Quickly, it became obvious that I took offense to how God was exposing me to His truth. I felt like I had been betrayed. Knowing God meant getting to know His heart and His dream for my life. His plan based on His terms. I began to see how I had expected God to bring my dreams to pass in the way that I had configured it in my head. I hadn't taken the time to ask Him what His dream was for me. I thought I already knew. I thought it had to be the same as mine!

After a while, the realization that I wasn't going to have my dreams come to pass the way I had anticipated was real. It literally felt like a death of a loved one. It was just that painful. Expectations are powerful, especially if they're deep rooted.

This is where the injury started. I began to speak of how regretful I was that I had given my life in service to God. It was my constant conversation to myself. I kept reliving the past like a broken record in my head. I kept trying to go back in my mind to redo the past.

We all know that no one can redo the past. Well, there's always the idea of the time machine where you go back in the past and redo the decision for a more favorable outcome. That's what I was trying so desperately to do, change the past in some way. Once again, I fell into a deep state of rebellion, despair, and regret. How foolish does that sound? But desperate times called for desperate measures (plain stupid, but real)! Regret had convinced me that talking about it all the time would somehow make a difference. Oh, it made a difference alright; and yes, that does mean I wasn't in my right mind.

In the midst of this devastation, the Lord challenged me to deal with my ego. During this time, the character "SheQuiQui" was brought into the light. She was my old, carnal self. She was the part of me that had dreamed, since the age of 9, of being someone significant in the world. I didn't want to serve the Lord anymore if it meant experiencing the loss of my dreams, on my terms. At that point, I was very willing to walk away from God and live like an unbeliever.

BUT GOD! He was faithful, and He still had His plan.

CHAPTER 10

Seven Ways God Wants Respect

How many of us think that we are disrespecting God? We know how we act when someone disrespects us. I had been studying the book of Romans for about 3 years. The Lord began to explain to me that He has His ways of wanting respect from the world and his people. When we disrespect God, He has consequences that are designed to teach us to respect Him, just as our parents did. In Romans 1:18–20, God talks about how the world disrespects Him:

For [God does not overlook sin and] the wrath of God is revealed from heaven against all ungodliness and unrighteousness of men who in their wickedness suppress and stifle the truth, because that which is known about God is evident within them [in their inner consciousness], for God made it evident to them. For ever since the creation of the world His invisible attributes, His eternal power and divine nature, have been clearly seen, being understood through His workmanship [all His creation, the wonderful things that He has made], so that they [who fail to believe and trust in Him] are without excuse and without defense.

Many Christians have been taught that the Lord is only talking about homosexuality, but He said all ungodliness and unrighteousness. He addresses the church folk in Romans 2: 5–10:

But because of your callous stubbornness and unrepentant heart you are [deliberately] storing up wrath for yourself on the day of wrath when God's righteous judgment will be revealed. He WILL PAY BACK TO EACH PERSON ACCORDING TO HIS DEEDS [justly, as his deeds deserve]: to those who by persistence in doing good seek [unseen but cer-

tain heavenly] glory, honor, and immortality, [He will give the gift of] eternal life. But for those who are selfishly ambitious and self-seeking and disobedient to the truth but responsive to wickedness, [there will be] wrath and indignation. There will be tribulation and anguish [torturing confinement] for every human soul who does [or permits] evil, to the Jew first and also to the Greek, but glory and honor and inner peace [will be given] to everyone who habitually does well, to the Jew first and also to the Greek. For God shows no partiality [no arbitrary favoritism; with Him one person isn't more important than another].

What does all this have to do with me? I had disrespected God in rejecting different parts of me. Our bodies, our emotions, our thoughts, and our egos are designed to serve the Lord, not to master us. Certain parts of me I accepted; certain parts I rejected. He wanted to teach me how to love myself, unconditionally, just as he does. Well, I didn't know how to do that.

The Lord had already been teaching and training me on how He wanted me to honor and respect Him through who I was as a person. He died for every part of me.

Romans 5:6–11 (JB)

And we can see that it was while we were powerless to help ourselves that Christ died for sinful men. In human experience it's a rare thing for one man to give his life for another, even if the latter be a good man, though there have been a few who have had the courage to do it. Yet the proof of God's amazing love is this: that it was while we were sinners that Christ died for us. Moreover, if he did that for us while we were sinners, now that we are men justified by the shedding of his blood, what reason have we to fear the wrath of God? If, while we were his enemies, Christ reconciled us to God by dying for us, surely now that we are reconciled we may be perfectly certain of our salvation through his living in us. Nor, I am sure, is this a matter of bare salvation—we may hold our heads high in the light of God's love because of the reconciliation which Christ has made

He had given me seven components of health that would help me measure how well I was respecting God the way He wanted to be respected: learning how to be still and listen, high octane nutrition, proper hydration, exercise/movement, stress management, supplementation, and balanced emotional health. It was the highest calling, loving every part of me, unconditionally. The cancer was speaking loud and clear on accepting every part of who I am, including my ego.

For many years I accepted the teaching that the old self was dead, no longer existed and had no value. We can never get rid of our history. Once we belong to Christ, our history is no longer supposed to controls us or defines us, but in the hands of God, it's used to bring glory to our God's transforming power. I had disrespected myself from God's perspective. So much self-denial, it was unbelievable. I thought this was an honorable thing in God's sight. I was so empty, so broken, and so miserable. Do we really want God's truth? Do we really want God's will? Or do we want God to bless what we want for His kingdom and label it for His purpose?

To be honest, I was a miserable Christian, constantly fighting myself. A war was going on inside me constantly! No more wars, praise the name of the living God! I walk free of guilt and condemnation because I've accepted my whole self as God is teaching me how. I didn't stop to ask God what death meant to Him. I just implemented my own definitions, which caused me a great deal of unhappiness and defeat. I kept asking God to tell me what I was missing on this Christian journey. When I read the Bible and I looked at my life, I saw a great discrepancy. Very little victory over sin, self, and Satan. The cancer forced me to acknowledge my history, my ego, my way of looking at life and God. When those health challenges came into my life, I felt like the circumstances said, "Will the real Japonica Rena Walker, please stand up?" and she did with a great roar! My "SheQuiQui" refused to be silenced any longer. There was no way I could shut her up anymore. God was demanding that I respect that part of me, because He paid a great price for my ego.

1 Corinthians 6:18–20 (NIRV) says:

Keep far away from sexual sins. All the other sins a person commits are outside the body. But sexual sins are sins against their own body. Don't you know that your bodies are temples of the Holy Spirit? The Spirit is in you, and you have received the Spirit from God. You do not belong to yourselves. Christ has paid the price for you. So use your bodies in a way that honors God.

As I spent time at the institute, the Lord continued to bring this memory, as well as others to mind. They began to flood my soul, my thoughts, my emotions, and my imagination. The entire experience absolutely blew my mind! He also continued to minister to me about the root of the cancer.

As the healing of my emotions progressed, He showed me a vision of my grandbaby falling down on her bike and injuring herself. I heard Him ask the question, "How would you help her? Would you chastise her to get up quickly and cut the wound out and off?" That seemed to be an obvious "No sir!" The concept penetrated my soul! It was then that the Lord began to teach me about the different types of injuries and their parallel to emotional wounds.

The first wound that He talked about was a scratch. Imagine one of your children when they were small. When they got a flesh wound, you were careful to administer some kind of care to reassure them of your love for them.

Next, He talked about a stab wound. This one was a little bit more severe than a scratch and would require some kind of assistance and more attention to details on the quality of care. It would take a little longer to heal than a scratch.

The last example he gave was that of a severe gunshot wound. In the natural world, a gunshot wound would require immediate medical attention. This isn't something we can handle ourselves. It would require professional help. Many times lifesaving surgery would be a must.

After God's explanation of the types of emotional wounds we could experience, I knew immediately what kind of wound I had suffered. For two years, I had allowed my regrets about obeying God to fester and cause sheer havoc! While I knew this principle to be true of forgiveness, I hadn't given a second thought to what the attitude of regret was doing. It began to make sense. Any emotion allowed to grow like the "Incredible Hulk" certainly has its own personality.

This trauma was a gunshot wound that had not been tended to. It was oozing with puss and many different types of infections! This severe wound manifested itself in my body as breast cancer. My body was doing all it could to tell me something was wrong, but it took breast cancer to get me to sit down and listen to what it had to say. It was demanding my attention.

Before moving on, let me clarify my position on my personal journey. Every person is different when it comes to diseases. This was my <u>personal</u> experience based on my desire to live in the face of crisis. A diagnosis of cancer is scary, regardless of what path is chosen.

I had a great desire to seek my Creator first; and then, incorporate whatever medical tools that would help me do what was best for me. This was the path He chose for me. My health status was going to be whatever I decided. I was willing to take the risk of trusting in my faith. Not everyone is at that place. I chose not to completely trust my life to another human being who knew nothing about me, or my body. As I sought the One whom I believed had the answers for my crisis, Jesus Christ, my Savior, I realized that my power lay in my ability to decide.

That being said, everyone has to choose their own path, especially when it comes to something like cancer. I'm certainly not insinuating that all diseases are created by our own hands; however, far too many of the diseases people are experiencing are preventable.

The biggest takeaway that I would love for people to see is that no matter what's going on in your life, if we ask God to teach us how to trust Him in situations that are extremely difficult, He will bring some good things out of the most difficult and life-changing problems as He promised in Romans 8:28–30:

> *Moreover, we know that to those who love God, who are called according to his plan, everything that happens fits into a pattern for good. God, in his foreknowledge, chose them to bear the family likeness of his Son, that he might be the eldest of a family of many brothers. He chose them long ago; when the time came he called them, he made them righteous in his sight, and then lifted them to the splendor of life as his own sons.*

STUDY GUIDE QUESTIONS

My Gift #1: Name a time that you prayed, and God answered it as a time of refining to develop holiness in you.

_____

_____

_____

_____

My Gift #2: Many times, I assumed that I knew how to trust God. It was imperative that I learn how to trust God in each situation, so I wouldn't fall prey to unrealized expectations (i.e., disappointment).

Name one area where you are struggling in knowing how to trust God.

_____

_____

_____

_____

_____

_____

CHAPTER 11

Getting to Know Him

During this harrowing trek, one of the things that I've learned about God is that He gets so excited when there are opportunities for us to learn to trust Him. These circumstances usually look like we have completely lost control in the natural realm.

It's so easy for us to pray to know Him, but do we really understand that life's problems constantly create an environment to trust in the living God? Do we really understand who we're praying to and that He hears every prayer and answers them, one way or the other, in His time?

I've learned and am still learning that this journey of trusting God through breast cancer has been a gift in so many ways. Maybe not from a worldly point of view, but certainly from a kingdom point of view.

In the beginning, I was terrified of this whole process. He taught me about myself and how much I disrespected who I was. Many ugly and unbelieving parts of me were called out into the light. Even when I couldn't stand all this ugliness, the Father showed me how to love and honor every ugly, disrespectful, and rebellious part.

I learned about my ego and that she was and still is a vital part of who I am. It was never God's intent for me to disregard any part of my human journey. He continues to use my 'humanness' for His Kingdom purposes. I learned that I am "three in one" just like the Holy Trinity. Certainly, I was created in His imagine. It all makes so much sense. NOW! If it weren't for this experience, I wouldn't have gotten to know SheQuiQui and Raynale (My ego and rational self). They're vital parts of my human team. They have a rightful place in the kingdom, and it's at the foot of the cross, not the throne of my life.

I now have a basic understanding of what Romans 7:14–25 mean when it talks about how my spiritual self and my ego were constantly fighting with each other:

We know that the Law is right and good, but I am a person who does what is wrong and bad. I am not my own boss. Sin is my boss. I do not understand myself. I want to do what is right but I do not do it. Instead, I do the very thing I hate. When I do the thing I do not want to do, it shows me that the Law is right and good. So I am not doing it. Sin living in me is doing it. I know There's nothing good in me, that is, in my flesh. For I want to do well but I do not. I do not do the good I want to do. Instead, I am always doing the sinful things I do not want to do. If I am always doing the very thing I do not want to do, it means I am no longer the one who does it. It's sin that lives in me. This has become my way of life: When I want to do what is right, I always do what is wrong. My mind and heart agree with the Law of God. But there's a different law at work deep inside of me that fights with my mind. This law of sin holds me in its power because sin is still in me. There's no happiness in me! Who can set me free from my sinful old self? God's Law has power over my mind, but sin still has power over my sinful old self.

I thank God that I can be free through Jesus Christ our Lord! I can and do declare that because of this journey, God has brought this internal war to an end! Only the God of the universe could set me free from that old self being in control. I am eternally grateful!

My relationship to God and people has been purified and become genuine and authentic. I can truly say it's been an awesome adventure, experiencing the God of the universe and what He is capable of doing in me and through me.

One of the things that God has said to me is, "I need my people to be willing to go into the darkness where people are hurting and bring them hope and bring them out of the darkness."

Our God is a God who loves people. Nothing is wasted in our lives. God isn't surprised by anything we encounter. I've been able to talk to people who've been diagnosed with some form of cancer and were scared just as I was. Because of the Lord Jesus Christ, I was able to provide hope and comfort. That doesn't mean that they didn't go through traditional treatment. What it means is that when I shared with them what I had learned, it gave them hope.

STUDY GUIDE QUESTIONS

My Gift #1: Will you willingly allow the Lord to take you into the dark room to develop His character in you and through you so that others might see hope?

_____

My Gift #2: Salvation is Free, but godly holiness costs! Worldly holiness and godly holiness are two different concepts. Look at Romans 1:4, Romans 6:19, and Romans 6:22 in three different translation.

My Gift #3: Unwrap your thoughts on Romans 1:4

_____

_____

_____

_____

_____

_____

_____

My Gift #4: Unwrap your thoughts on Romans 6:19

_____

_____

_____

_____

_____

_____

_____

_____

My Gift #5. Unwrap your thoughts on Romans 6:22

_____

_____

_____

_____

_____

_____

_____

_____

ADDITIONAL STUDY QUESTIONS

My Gift #1: Research has shown that our lifestyles, nutrition, lack of water, lack of exercise, stress, and relationship breakdowns contributes greatly to immune dysfunction and compromise. When the immune system is weakened, we are vulnerable to anything.

Meditation:

_____

_____

_____

_____

_____

_____

My Gift #2: Studies have proven that getting adequate sleep is instrumental in health, weight loss, and minimizing stress. Take some time to pay attention to how well you're sleeping. Note how much sleep you're getting and where you can make some improvements.

Benefits of good sleep: helps the body to repair, resets the metabolism, reduces stress, helps with weight loss, and improves memory.

Sleep:

_____

_____

_____

_____

_____

_____

My Gift #3: Benefits of all forms of nutrition: better mood, cellular respect and reparation, improved mood, diminished internal conflict, reduced emotional eating, and weight loss.

Nutrition:

    a. Words/self-talk/thoughts:
    b. Emotions:
    c. Relationships:
    d. Food Choices:

_____

_____

_____

_____

_____

_____

_____

My Gift # 4: The human body has been reported to be approximately 60–75% water. Several studies have indicated that average human can go up to 21 days without food and survive. However, hydration is a different story. Typically, the average person can go only about 3–4 days without water before endangering their life. Good old-fashioned water is good for general health.

A good way to measure if your body is getting enough water is to take your present weight, divide it in half. This number as ounces is a great indicator of how much water you should be taking in. No less than! If you find water to be a struggle, start with where you are now and start building to get your destination.

Benefits: regulates body temperature, lubricates joints, helps prevent constipation, carries nutrients and oxygen to cells, promotes weight loss, fights infections, boosts energy, and reduces the risk of cancer.

Example: If you drink 20 ounces, start drinking 20 ounces for 7–10 days (listen to your body). Consistency is the key.

Hydration:

1st 7–10 days: 20 ounces of water:

2nd 7–10 days: add 8–16 ounces of water to the 20 ounces total 28–26 ounces (be consistent)

3rd 7–10 days: add another 8–16 ounces of water to the 28–36 ounces of water (be consistent)

You can certainly add more water if needed, but you certainly you don't want to do any less than what is planned out for that week. Be creative! Add fruit or veggies to enhance the water if it makes it easier to drink.

You keep adding on to the previous week until you reach your goal. Now of course, all of this will vary based on the person, so I encourage you not to use these guidelines as a law, but a tool to help to establish some sound and healthy tools for your body.

Never make the plan more important than the person. Keep yourself as a priority!

_____

_____

_____

_____

_____

_____

_____

My Gift #5: There are so many benefits to different forms of exercising. Choose the form you feel most comfortable with. You always want to check with your Healthcare provider whenever a change is being made in your life, so that you remain safe and on the same page as your healthcare team.

You are the captain of your healthcare, so never give away your power to decide about your health but always use wisdom in how to communicate with your team.

Benefits: good for muscles and bones, brain health and memory, helps to reduce chronic diseases, increase energy levels, helps with emotional stability, and aids in weight loss.

Physical Exercise/Movement: Mark where you are. Start there!

General Guidelines:

Beginner Level: 15–30 minutes of light exercise 1–3 times a week (at least 2 days of rest from exercise)

General Population Level: at least 30 minutes of moderate exercise 4–5 times a week (at least 2 days of rest from exercise)

Intermediate Level: at least 60 minutes of vigorous exercise 4–5 times a week (at least 2 days of rest from exercise)

Advance Level: at least 60–90 minutes of vigorous of cross-training exercise 5–6 times a week (include at least one day of rest per week from exercise)

_____

_____

_____

_____

_____

_____

_____

My Gift #6: During our busy lives, supplementation is necessary. The quality of our foods have diminished and most of us live a pretty fast-paced life where fast foods are a part of our lifestyle. An overall good multivitamin is something we can all benefit from, so start there first. A multivitamin will help provide what you may not be getting from your food. Shop around! Plenty of options are available.

Benefits: addresses general dietary deficiencies, helps eliminate toxins from the body, supports healthy aging, helps increase bowel movements, helps to build the immune system, helps with the metabolism, and aids in weight loss.

Supplementations:

Multivitamins—one that will provide at least 100% of the Daily Vitamins for at least 13 vitamins

Food Enzymes—provides a blend of enzymes to digest proteins, carbohydrates, and fats.

B-Complex—any formula that will support the nervous system

_____

_____

_____

_____

_____

_____

_____

My Gift #7: Proper elimination is the last of my seven components. Please don't be mistaken; it's not the least of the seven. In my personal and professional opinion, it's the most important of all! Do your research! Gut health is vital to health and wellness. If "your trash" is piling up in the "house," somebody is going to have to take it out! Respect the function of your colon! Benefits: removing waste, aids in elimination of toxins from the body, important for brain and emotional health, reduces the risk of cancer.

Bowel Movements: According to naturopathy, a healthy body will eliminate after each major meal. At least one bowel movement per day is recommended as a good starting place.

If you are dealing with elimination issues, I recommend that you speak to a natural healthcare provider or a functional medical doctor.

_____

_____

_____

_____

_____

_____

_____

_____

_____

Resources

Biblegateway.com

The Molecules of Emotions—Candace Pert, PhD

Feelings Buried Alive Never Die—Karol Truman

The C Word Movie—featuring Dr. David Servan-Schreiber and narrated by Morgan Freeman

The Biology of Belief—Bruce Lipton, PhD

The Living Matrix Documentary

Optimum Health Institute—http://www.optimumhealth.org

A Cancer Battle Plan—Anne E. Frahm, David J. Frahm

Never Be Sick Again— Raymond Francis

www.ingramcontent.com/pod-product-compliance
Lightning Source LLC
Chambersburg PA
CBHW060515280326
41933CB00014B/2977